CHIROPRACTIC TECHNIQUES FOR BEGINNERS

Step-By-Step Instructions And Essential Tips To Improve Spinal Health, Relieve Pain, And Enhance Well-Being

DR SAWYER DIEGO

Copyright © [2024] by [Dr. .Sawyer Diego]. All rights reserved.

Except for brief quotations included in critical reviews and certain other noncommercial uses allowed by copyright law, no part of this publication may be reproduced, distributed, or transmitted in any form or by any means, including photocopying, recording, or other electronic or mechanical methods, without the publisher's prior written permission.

DISCLAMER

Nothing in this book should be interpreted as medical advice; it is meant exclusively for educational reasons. Regarding their specific health issues and treatment options, readers are urged to speak with licensed healthcare professionals. The publisher and author disclaim all liability for any errors or omissions in the material provided, as well as for any negative effects that may arise from using or abusing the information. Although every attempt has been taken to guarantee that the material in this book is correct as of the date of publishing, new research may have superseded some of the content because medical knowledge is always changing. It is recommended that readers confirm the most recent medical recommendations and guidelines. The reader of this book undertakes to release the author and publisher from any claims or liabilities resulting from the use of this information, and understands and accepts the inherent risks connected with healthcare decisions.

TABLE OF CONTENTS

CHAPTER ONE 11
CHIROPRACTIC TECHNIQUES OVERVIEW 11
- CHIROPRACTIC CARE: WHAT IS IT? 11
- ADVANTAGES OF CHIROPRACTIC METHODS 13
- SAFETY POINTS TO REMEMBER 14
- HOW TO MAKE THE MOST OF THIS BOOK 17
- AN OVERVIEW OF FREQUENTLY USED TERMINOLOGIES IN 19

CHAPTER TWO 21
COMPREHENDING CHIROPRACTIC CARE 21
- CHIROPRACTIC: DEFINITION AND BACKGROUND 21
- THE PHILOSOPHY AND GUIDING PRINCIPLES OF CHIROPRACTIC 23
- PRACTICE AREA COVERAGE AND LEGAL ISSUES 25
- CHIROPRACTIC AND CONVENTIONAL MEDICINE DISTINCTIONS 26
- THE VALUE OF PROPER SPINAL ALIGNMENT AND HEALTH 28

CHAPTER THREE 31
FUNDAMENTALS OF SPINAL ANATOMY 31
- THE SPINE'S STRUCTURE AND FUNCTION 31
- AN OVERVIEW OF DISCS AND VERTEBRAE 32
- THE VALUE OF PROPER SPINAL ALIGNMENT 34
- COMMON SPINAL CONDITIONS THAT CHIROPRACTIC CARE 35

CHAPTER FOUR 39
FIRST CHIROPRACTIC EXAM 39
- THE INITIAL CONSULTATION'S GOAL 39
- COMPREHENSIVE MEDICAL HISTORY AND EVALUATION 40

- METHODS OF PHYSICAL EXAMINATION EMPLOYED BY 42
- IMAGING DIAGNOSTICS AND ADDITIONAL DIAGNOSTIC 43
- CREATING PRACTICAL THERAPY OBJECTIVES 45

CHAPTER FIVE 47
- TECHNIQUES FOR ADJUSTMENTS IN CHIROPRACTIC 47
  - THE PURPOSE AND DEFINITION OF CHIROPRACTIC ADJUSTMENTS .. 47
  - VARIOUS ADJUSTMENT TECHNIQUE TYPES 49
  - PRACTICAL DISPLAY OF ADJUSTMENT PROCESSES 50
  - SAFETY OBSERVATIONS WHEN MAKING CHANGES 52
  - SUBSEQUENT CARE FOLLOWING ADJUSTMENTS 54

CHAPTER SIX 57
- ADJUNCTIVE THERAPIES IN CHIROPRACTIC MEDICINE 57
  - SYNOPSIS OF COMPLEMENTARY MEDICINE 57
  - HOW CHIROPRACTIC ADJUSTMENTS ARE SUPPORTED BY 58
  - ADVANTAGES AND DRAWBACKS OF EVERY THERAPY 59
  - COMBINING THERAPIES FOR ALL-INCLUSIVE CARE 61
  - TAILORED CARE PROGRAMS 62

CHAPTER SEVEN 65
- CONDITIONS CHIROPRACTORS TREAT 65
  - TREATMENT FOR COMMON MUSCULOSKELETAL CONDITIONS 65
  - CHIROPRACTIC BENEFITS FOR PARTICULAR CONDITIONS 66
  - EVIDENCE-BASED CHIROPRACTIC CARE METHODS 67
  - CASE STUDIES SHOWING EFFECTIVE THERAPIES 68
  - THE VALUE OF CONTINUOUS CHIROPRACTIC CARE FOR LONG-TERM ILLNESSES 70

CHAPTER EIGHT 71
THE RISKS AND SAFETY OF CHIROPRACTIC CARE 71
RECOGNIZING THE SAFETY PROFILE OF CHIROPRACTIC ADJUSTMENT METHODS 71
HAZARDS ASSOCIATED WITH ADJUSTMENTS IN CHIROPRACTIC 73
PRECAUTIONS FOR PATIENT POPULATIONS AT HIGH RISK 74
HOW TO PICK A REPUTABLE CHIROPRACTOR 76
LEGAL AND MORAL ISSUES IN THE PRACTICE OF CHIROPRACTIC 77

CHAPTER NINE 79
COMBINING CHIROPRACTIC THERAPY WITH OTHER MEDICAL SPECIALTIES 79
WORKING COOPERATIVELY WITH PHYSICIANS AND SPECIALISTS 79
MULTIDISCIPLINARY COMMUNICATION'S SIGNIFICANCE 81
WHEN TO SEND PATIENTS TO DIFFERENT MEDICAL 82
CHIROPRACTIC'S PLACE IN INTEGRATIVE HEALTH 84
PATIENT INSTRUCTION REGARDING COMBINATION THERAPY 86

CHAPTER TEN 89
CHANGES IN LIFESTYLE FOR SPINAL HEALTH 89
THE VALUE OF ERGONOMICS AND POSTURE 89
TIPS FOR CREATING AN ERGONOMIC WORK AND HOME 90
INCLUDING STRETCHING AND EXERCISE PROGRAMS 92
DIETARY SUGGESTIONS TO PROMOTE SPINAL HEALTH 93
THE EFFECTS OF STRESS MANAGEMENT STRATEGIES ON 94

CHAPTER ELEVEN 97
FAQS & FREQUENTLY ASKED QUESTIONS 97

COMMON QUESTIONS AND ANSWERS REGARDING CHIROPRACTIC CARE 97

RESOLVING SAFETY AND EFFECTIVENESS ISSUES................................99

WHAT TO ANTICIPATE FROM A VISIT TO THE CHIROPRACTOR........101

HOW TO LOCATE A TRUSTWORTHY CHIROPRACTOR 103

SOURCES OF ADDITIONAL DATA AND ASSISTANCE 105

ABOUT THE BOOK

"Chiropractic Techniques for Beginners" is a vital resource for anyone who wants to know how to use and benefit from chiropractic care. It starts by demystifying chiropractic care, describing its history, and highlighting its basic principles. It also makes clear the differences between chiropractic and conventional medicine, highlighting the critical role that spinal health plays in overall health. Knowledge of spinal anatomy is important because it lays the groundwork for understanding the various chiropractic techniques that chiropractors use to optimize spinal alignment and function. Finally, the book thoroughly covers common spinal conditions that chiropractors treat, emphasizing the direct relationship between spinal health and overall health.

A salient aspect of this manual is its thorough examination of the first chiropractic examination process. Readers learn about the intent behind consultations, the value of patient history, and the variety of diagnostic instruments that chiropractors use. Hands-on examples of chiropractic adjustment techniques, like activators and diversified methods, guarantee that readers understand the objectives and safety concerns of the procedures. The incorporation of supplemental therapies, like therapeutic exercises and ultrasound, augments the efficacy of chiropractic care and promotes individualized treatment regimens.

Along with a thorough discussion of safety in chiropractic care, the book also explores evidence-based approaches to treating musculoskeletal conditions such as sciatica and back pain, bolstered by compelling case studies that demonstrate successful outcomes. The guide also advocates for collaborative healthcare approaches, highlighting the significance of interdisciplinary communication and knowing when to refer patients to other specialists. Finally, safety in chiropractic care is thoroughly covered.

The book also includes a thorough discussion of lifestyle changes that support spinal health, such as ergonomics, stress management, and posture tips. Common questions about chiropractic care are answered in the FAQ section, which also offers advice on choosing reputable chiropractors. Throughout, the book encourages readers to take an active role in their journey toward spinal health by providing helpful resources for more information and support.

By bridging the gap between theory and practice, "Chiropractic Techniques for Beginners" stands out as an extensive resource that gives readers the knowledge necessary to make informed decisions about their health and well-being. It also gives beginners the tools they need to navigate chiropractic care with confidence and effectiveness.

CHAPTER ONE

CHIROPRACTIC TECHNIQUES OVERVIEW

CHIROPRACTIC CARE: WHAT IS IT?

Chiropractic care is a holistic approach to health that focuses on the musculoskeletal system, particularly the spine. The fundamental idea behind chiropractic treatment is that the body can heal itself without the need for medication or surgery if the spine is properly aligned. Trained in this area, chiropractors use hands-on spinal manipulation and other alternative therapies to improve mobility, relieve pain, and support the body's natural healing process.

By making adjustments and manipulating the spine, chiropractors hope to restore alignment and relieve pressure on nerves, which can improve overall health and wellness. Many patients seek chiropractic care for conditions like joint problems, back pain, and neck pain. The practice emphasizes the significance of maintaining proper spinal alignment.

Chiropractors use their hands or specialized instruments to apply controlled force to the affected joints, aiming to restore alignment and mobility. Treatment plans are customized to each patient's specific needs and may include adjustments, therapeutic exercises, and ergonomic advice. Chiropractic care is not just about treating symptoms but also about addressing underlying causes to promote long-term health and wellness. It is considered a safe and effective treatment option for many musculoskeletal conditions, often integrated with conventional medicine.

In addition to focusing on preventive care to maintain spinal health and overall well-being, chiropractic adjustments frequently provide patients with pain relief and improved mobility.

Regular visits to the chiropractor can also help prevent injuries, improve posture, and enhance athletic performance. Some chiropractors also provide lifestyle advice and nutritional counseling to support holistic health.

Overall, chiropractic care focuses on restoring balance within the body to facilitate natural healing processes and improve quality of life.

ADVANTAGES OF CHIROPRACTIC METHODS

Many patients find that chiropractic care relieves pain without the need for medications or invasive procedures, making it a preferred option for that seeking drug-free pain management. One of the main benefits of chiropractic techniques is pain relief, especially for conditions affecting the spine, such as lower back pain and neck discomfort.

Through spinal adjustments, chiropractors can relieve pressure on nerves and reduce inflammation, which often leads to significant pain reduction.

Chiropractic adjustments support immune function by removing interference to the nervous system, which is crucial for immune response and overall health maintenance. In addition to relieving pain, chiropractic care promotes overall wellness by improving nervous system communication and spinal function. Proper spinal alignment increases mobility and flexibility, allowing the body to move more efficiently and with less discomfort, which can benefit athletes and individuals with active lifestyles by optimizing performance and reducing the risk of injuries.

Chiropractors help restore bodily balance by correcting misaligned spines, which can enhance digestion, mental clarity, and sleep quality. Many patients experience an overall improvement in their quality of life after receiving chiropractic care, as it supports the body's natural healing abilities and promotes long-term health benefits. This is just one of the many noteworthy benefits of chiropractic techniques, which go beyond simply treating symptoms.

SAFETY POINTS TO REMEMBER

As with any medical or therapeutic intervention, there are some safety precautions to take into account when receiving chiropractic care. Firstly, make sure the chiropractor you choose is qualified, having completed accredited training and holding a license to practice in your state or nation.

This guarantees that the practitioner has the knowledge and skills necessary to perform spinal adjustments safely and effectively.

To create a customized treatment plan that meets your individual needs and concerns, you must have an extensive assessment and evaluation performed by your chiropractor before receiving chiropractic treatment.

This evaluation should cover your medical history, current symptoms, and any pre-existing health conditions. You should also be transparent with your chiropractor regarding any pain or discomfort you may be experiencing during or after treatment, as well as any concerns you may have regarding the techniques being used.

While some patients may experience mild soreness or stiffness following chiropractic adjustments, this usually resolves within a day or two. Serious complications from chiropractic care are rare but can include nerve injury or worsened pain if adjustments are not performed correctly. Popping or cracking sounds are normal during spinal adjustments and are caused by the release of gas bubbles within the joint. This is a natural and harmless phenomenon.

You can safely experience the potential health and well-being benefits of chiropractic care by selecting a qualified chiropractor and remaining informed about the process. To ensure safety during chiropractic treatment, it's essential to follow your chiropractor's recommendations regarding the frequency of visits and any additional therapies or exercises prescribed. If you have any concerns about the safety of chiropractic techniques, discuss them with your healthcare provider before beginning treatment.

HOW TO MAKE THE MOST OF THIS BOOK

To fully benefit from this book on chiropractic techniques for beginners, you must be open-minded and eager to learn about holistic health practices. To start, familiarize yourself with the fundamentals of chiropractic care, including its benefits and guiding principles.

Take note of the way the book is organized, as it will walk you through each concept step-by-step, from understanding spinal alignment to using adjustments practically.

Make sure you go over any diagrams or illustrations included in the book; they can help you better understand intricate anatomical concepts and adjustment techniques.

As you read each chapter, make notes and highlight any points that speak to you. This will help you retain your understanding of chiropractic techniques and how they might affect your health.

Apply what you learn to real-world situations to engage with the material actively. Think about how you can incorporate the principles of chiropractic into your daily routine to support overall health and avoid musculoskeletal problems. If at all possible, talk with a licensed chiropractor or healthcare provider about your reading to get more clarification on any concepts you may not understand or to ask any questions you may have about specific techniques or terminology.

Finally, in your journey with chiropractic care, stay committed to lifelong learning and personal growth. Keep up with the latest findings, innovative treatment methods, and useful advice for preserving spinal health.

By effectively utilizing this book as a resource and educational tool, you will equip yourself to make well-informed decisions about your health and investigate the potential advantages of chiropractic techniques for long-term wellness.

AN OVERVIEW OF FREQUENTLY USED TERMINOLOGIES IN CHIROPRACTIC

To communicate with patients and colleagues in the field of chiropractic care, one must be familiar with several technical terms and concepts that are essential to the field. One such term is "subluxation," which describes a misalignment of the vertebrae in the spine that can impair nerve function and general health. Subluxations are treated by chiropractors through adjustments or manipulations to realign the spine properly and relieve related symptoms.

The application of controlled force to the spine or joints to improve mobility and relieve pain is known as "spinal manipulation," and it is a key component of chiropractic treatments. To support long-term spinal health, this technique is frequently combined with therapeutic exercises and ergonomic advice. Patients who are aware of these terms are better able to participate in their treatment plans and communicate effectively with their chiropractors regarding their health goals and concerns.

Furthermore, before beginning treatment, chiropractors may use diagnostic instruments like "x-rays" to evaluate spinal alignment and pinpoint problem areas. X-rays offer important information about the structural integrity of the spine and assist chiropractors in customizing adjustments to each patient's unique needs. Patients can make educated decisions about their healthcare and feel comfortable interacting with chiropractors by being familiar with common terminology and procedures.

CHAPTER TWO
COMPREHENDING CHIROPRACTIC CARE

CHIROPRACTIC: DEFINITION AND BACKGROUND

Chiropractic care is a branch of medicine that focuses on the diagnosis, treatment, and prevention of mechanical disorders of the musculoskeletal system, especially the spine. It highlights the connection between the structure and function of the body.

The first chiropractic adjustment was made in 1895 by D.D. Palmer, who is sometimes credited with founding the field. Since then, chiropractic has developed into a globally recognized healthcare profession. Its basic tenet is that when the musculoskeletal system, especially the spine, is properly aligned, the body can heal itself without the need for surgery or medication, improving overall health and well-being.

The field of chiropractic care has expanded to include various specialized techniques and approaches tailored to individual patient needs, making chiropractic care accessible to a wide range of health conditions beyond just spinal issues.

Typically, chiropractic techniques involve manual manipulation or adjustments of the spine or other joints to correct misalignments, known as subluxations that can cause pain, discomfort, or hinder normal function. These adjustments are often accompanied by other treatments like exercises, stretches, and lifestyle counseling to support the body's natural healing process.

To address the underlying causes of musculoskeletal issues through precise adjustments and supportive therapies, chiropractic aims to restore proper function, alleviate pain, and improve the overall quality of life for patients of all ages. Therefore, understanding the historical roots and modern applications of chiropractic is crucial for both practitioners and patients seeking non-invasive, holistic approaches to health and wellness.

THE PHILOSOPHY AND GUIDING PRINCIPLES OF CHIROPRACTIC TECHNIQUES

The foundational ideas of chiropractic philosophy and techniques stem from multiple core beliefs that inform chiropractic practice. First, the idea that the body has a natural capacity to heal itself when the nervous system is operating at peak performance is central to chiropractic philosophy. This belief is consistent with the notion that the structural integrity of the spine directly affects the body's overall health and well-being. Secondly, chiropractors emphasize the importance of maintaining proper spinal alignment to ensure the nervous system can effectively transmit signals, which in turn facilitates healing and maintains optimal health.

The foundation of chiropractic care is the idea that spinal misalignments, or subluxations, can impair nerve function and interfere with the body's natural healing processes. By making precise adjustments, chiropractors seek to correct these misalignments, restoring proper nerve function and fostering overall wellness.

There is a wide range of techniques used by chiropractors, from manual adjustments to more modern methods that use specialized instruments or gentle, low-force techniques appropriate for patients of all ages and conditions.

Following these fundamental guidelines allows chiropractors to treat patients' symptoms as well as their underlying causes, resulting in long-term health benefits that go beyond short-term pain relief. This all-encompassing approach places a strong emphasis on patient education, lifestyle changes, and preventive care, enabling people to take charge of their health.

PRACTICE AREA COVERAGE AND LEGAL ISSUES

Chiropractors receive extensive education and training to diagnose, treat, and manage conditions related to spinal misalignments and joint dysfunctions. Their scope of practice includes performing manual adjustments, prescribing therapeutic exercises, offering nutritional advice, and providing lifestyle counseling to improve patient outcomes. The scope of chiropractic practice is broad and includes a wide range of musculoskeletal conditions, with a primary focus on the spine and its impact on overall health.

Chiropractic professionals must abide by state or provincial regulations and maintain compliance with professional ethics and standards. This guarantees that patients receive safe, effective care and have access to appropriate treatments within the scope of chiropractic practice. Legal considerations in chiropractic practice vary by jurisdiction.

Chiropractic care also requires collaboration with other healthcare providers, particularly when handling complex cases or sending patients for complementary treatments. Chiropractors can provide comprehensive care that meets the various needs of patients looking for non-conventional medical treatments by collaborating with medical doctors, physical therapists, and other healthcare professionals.

CHIROPRACTIC AND CONVENTIONAL MEDICINE DISTINCTIONS

Chiropractors view health through the lens of the alignment of the musculoskeletal system and its impact on overall wellness, whereas medical doctors approach health from a broader perspective that includes biochemical and physiological aspects of disease. Chiropractic and conventional medicine differ significantly in their approaches to healthcare and treatment modalities. While conventional medicine focuses on diagnosing and treating diseases using pharmaceuticals, surgery, and other interventions, chiropractic emphasizes natural healing methods and non-invasive techniques.

In contrast to conventional medicine, which primarily uses drugs, surgery, and diagnostic imaging to treat medical conditions based on scientific research and clinical trials, chiropractic care frequently uses manual adjustments to correct spinal misalignments and improve nervous system function. These adjustments are intended to restore mobility, alleviate pain, and enhance the body's ability to heal itself.

Despite these distinctions, the complementary roles that chiropractic and conventional medicine can play in integrated healthcare approaches are becoming more widely acknowledged. While many patients seek conventional medical treatments for acute illnesses and chronic conditions, chiropractic care is sought for musculoskeletal issues, pain management, and preventive health maintenance. This integrative approach enables patients to receive personalized care plans that address both short-term health concerns and long-term wellness goals.

THE VALUE OF PROPER SPINAL ALIGNMENT AND HEALTH

Achieving proper spinal alignment guarantees that nerve signals can travel unhindered between the brain and the rest of the body, facilitating communication that controls movement, sensation, and organ function. The importance of spinal health and alignment in chiropractic care cannot be overstated. The spine acts as the central support structure of the body, housing and protecting the spinal cord, which is essential to the nervous system's function.

A misaligned spine can result in a variety of health problems, such as musculoskeletal pain, decreased mobility, and impaired organ function due to nerve compression or interference. Chiropractors use specific techniques to correct these misalignments, relieving pressure on nerves and promoting the body's natural healing processes. Maintaining spinal health through chiropractic adjustments promotes optimal nerve function and enhances overall health and well-being.

Regular chiropractic care helps people of all ages maintain spinal health, improve posture, and lower the risk of chronic conditions associated with spinal dysfunction. By addressing spinal alignment proactively, chiropractors empower patients to enjoy better overall health outcomes and a higher quality of life through enhanced spinal function and nervous system integrity. In addition to providing pain relief, spinal alignment plays a crucial role in preventing future injuries and maintaining mobility as people age.

CHAPTER THREE

FUNDAMENTALS OF SPINAL ANATOMY

THE SPINE'S STRUCTURE AND FUNCTION

The spine also referred to as the vertebral column or backbone, is an essential anatomical structure in humans that offers protection, flexibility, and support. It is made up of 33 interlocking vertebrae arranged in five regions: the cervical (the neck), thoracic (the upper back), lumbar (the lower back), sacrum, and coccyx. Intervertebral discs serve as shock absorbers between the vertebrae and permit movement between them. The spine is surrounded by muscles and ligaments that provide stability and allow for a variety of movements, including bending, twisting, and extending.

Proper spinal alignment is essential for maintaining balance, preventing injuries, and supporting optimal nervous system function. The spine supports the body's weight and helps maintain an upright posture.

It also protects the spinal cord, a bundle of nerves that runs through the spinal canal formed by the vertebrae and transmits signals between the brain and the rest of the body, controlling movement, sensation, and bodily functions.

Chiropractic care is based on an understanding of the structure and function of the spine. Chiropractors emphasize the relationship between the nervous system and the spine, believing that spinal misalignments (subluxations) can affect overall health by interfering with nerve signals. Their goal is to restore proper alignment and function of the spine through manipulations and adjustments, thereby improving health and well-being.

AN OVERVIEW OF DISCS AND VERTEBRAE

The vertebrae, which are the building blocks of the spine, are each uniquely shaped to provide specific functions within different regions of the spinal column. The largest and strongest vertebrae support the body's weight and facilitate bending and lifting movements; the sacrum and coccyx at the base of the spine form a triangular structure, connecting the spine to the pelvis and providing stability; and the cervical vertebrae, located in the neck, support the head's weight and allow for neck movement. Thoracic vertebrae connect to the ribs and protect the chest's organs.

Chiropractic care often addresses disc-related issues through techniques that aim to reduce pressure on the discs and promote healing. Intervertebral discs are fibrocartilage structures that act as cushions and shock absorbers and are located between each vertebra. They are composed of an outer layer that is tough (annulus fibrosus) and an inner core that is gel-like (nucleus pulposus). These discs support the flexibility of the spine and allow for movements such as bending and twisting. Over time, discs can degenerate or herniate, causing pain and affecting spinal function.

To properly diagnose and treat spinal conditions, chiropractors must have a thorough understanding of the vertebrae and discs. By evaluating the health of the intervertebral discs and the condition of each vertebra, they can create individualized treatment plans that will relieve pain and restore spinal alignment.

THE VALUE OF PROPER SPINAL ALIGNMENT

An individual's posture, injury, or repeated stress can cause misalignment of the spine, which can result in subluxations (partial dislocations) that impair nerve function and overall health.

Spinal alignment, on the other hand, refers to the proper positioning of the vertebrae, ensuring that the spine maintains its natural curvature and functions optimally.

To maintain a healthy nervous system, misalignments can put pressure on nerves, resulting in pain, stiffness, and decreased mobility. Chiropractors use spinal adjustments to correct misalignments and restore proper nerve function, which not only relieves symptoms but also improves the body's natural healing capacity.

Spinal alignment is critical for long-term health and injury prevention. It supports healthy posture, lowers the risk of musculoskeletal disorders, and improves the body's adaptability to physical stressors.

The goals of chiropractic care are to improve spinal alignment through manual adjustments, specific exercises, and ergonomic recommendations for each patient.

COMMON SPINAL CONDITIONS THAT CHIROPRACTIC CARE CAN TREAT

Many spinal problems affecting the vertebrae, discs, and surrounding structures are frequently treated by chiropractors. These conditions include:

1. Subluxations: Modest misalignments of the vertebrae that might impede nerve transmission and result in discomfort.

2. Herniated discs occur when an intervertebral disc's inner core pushes through its outer shell, possibly squeezing spinal nerves and producing discomfort or weakness.

3. Degenerative Disc Disease: Pain, stiffness, and decreased flexibility are caused by the intervertebral discs gradually deteriorating over time.

4. Sciatica: compression of the sciatic nerve, usually resulting in discomfort extending down one leg from the lower back through the buttocks.

5. Spinal Stenosis: A narrowing of the spinal canal that can cause pain, numbness, or weakness by applying pressure to the spinal cord and nerves.

Chiropractors repair spinal irregularities to assist in alleviating pain and enhance general spine function. Their adjustments are intended to address these issues by restoring spinal alignment, minimizing nerve compression, and facilitating healing.

The Effects of Spinal Health on General Well-Being

An individual's overall well-being is greatly impacted by their state of spinal health. The nervous system function is optimally supported by a healthy spine, which facilitates effective communication between the brain and the body. This communication improves balance, coordination, and sensory perception.

A well-aligned spine lowers the risk of musculoskeletal pain and injuries; it also promotes healthy posture, which can ward off chronic conditions like headaches, and neck and back pain; it increases joint flexibility and mobility, which boosts general physical function and lowers the risk of injury during physical activity.

In addition to physical health, the alignment of the spine has an impact on mental and emotional health. Prolonged discomfort resulting from misaligned spines can cause stress, anxiety, and depression. By treating spinal problems with chiropractic adjustments, people can feel happier, sleep better, and have a higher quality of life overall.

Chiropractic adjustments, proper posture, and healthy lifestyle choices all contribute to maintaining spinal health, which is crucial for optimizing overall well-being. As practitioners of the holistic approach to health, they recognize the interdependence of spinal health and optimal bodily function.

CHAPTER FOUR

FIRST CHIROPRACTIC EXAM

THE INITIAL CONSULTATION'S GOAL

In chiropractic care, the first consultation is crucial to comprehending the patient's health concerns and developing a customized treatment plan. The process starts with creating a warm and inviting environment in which the chiropractor carefully listens to the patient's medical history, current symptoms, and lifestyle factors that may have an impact on their health.

This thorough evaluation enables the chiropractor to identify the underlying causes of the patient's discomfort or dysfunction, whether they are related to joint problems, muscular tension, or spinal misalignment.

In this session, the patient's goals for treatment—such as pain relief, increased mobility, or improved overall wellness—are discussed.

The chiropractor emphasizes holistic approaches to health that prioritize natural healing and spinal alignment. By encouraging open communication, the patient feels empowered and informed about their treatment journey.

In conclusion, the initial consultation establishes a thorough understanding of the patient's health history, concerns, and treatment goals, laying the groundwork for successful chiropractic interventions catered to their particular needs. It also sets the stage for a collaborative partnership between the chiropractor and the patient, focused on achieving optimal health outcomes through personalized care strategies.

COMPREHENSIVE MEDICAL HISTORY AND EVALUATION

A comprehensive patient history and health assessment is an essential part of the initial chiropractic consultation. It entails collecting detailed information about the patient's medical history, including prior injuries, surgeries, chronic conditions, and family medical history. Knowing these details enables the chiropractor to determine potential causes of pain or dysfunction and develop a treatment plan that is tailored to the patient's needs.

Beyond the patient's medical history, lifestyle factors like nutrition, exercise routines, posture, and stress levels are also included in the health assessment. These factors offer important insights into the patient's general health and help create a comprehensive understanding of their overall well-being.

The chiropractor makes sure that no detail is missed by actively listening to questions and making sure to ask thoughtful questions.

In conclusion, the thorough patient history and health evaluation allow the chiropractor to obtain relevant data necessary for accurately diagnosing and treating musculoskeletal problems. By looking at lifestyle and medical aspects of the patient's health, the chiropractor obtains a comprehensive understanding of the patient's condition, allowing for individualized treatment that targets the underlying causes of pain or discomfort.

METHODS OF PHYSICAL EXAMINATION EMPLOYED BY CHIROPRACTORS

From hands-on evaluations and specialized tests, chiropractors assess spinal alignment and identify any abnormalities that may be contributing to the patient's symptoms.

Chiropractors use a variety of physical examination techniques to assess musculoskeletal function and identify areas of concern. These techniques may include assessing posture, range of motion, joint mobility, muscle strength, and neurological function.

Additionally, orthopedic tests and neurological assessments may be performed to further evaluate the patient's musculoskeletal and nervous system function. Palpation is a primary technique used by chiropractors to feel for muscle tension, joint stiffness, or misalignments in the spine or extremities. This tactile assessment helps pinpoint areas of pain or restricted movement, guiding the chiropractor in developing targeted treatment strategies.

In conclusion, the physical examination methods employed by chiropractors play a critical role in the diagnosis of musculoskeletal disorders and the evaluation of overall spinal health. Using manual assessments and specialized tests, the chiropractor obtains vital data that guide treatment choices and facilitates the best possible musculoskeletal function.

IMAGING DIAGNOSTICS AND ADDITIONAL DIAGNOSTIC INSTRUMENTS

X-rays, MRIs, and CT scans are examples of diagnostic imaging that may be required in some circumstances to supplement the results of a physical examination. These imaging modalities offer detailed views of the spine, joints, and surrounding tissues, providing important information about any structural abnormalities, fractures, or degenerative changes that may call for particular treatment strategies.

To assess muscle activity, nerve function, and thermal patterns, chiropractors may also employ additional diagnostic tools like thermography, surface electromyography (EMG), or posture analysis software.

These tools aid in identifying areas of dysfunction that may not be evident through physical examination alone and help the chiropractor create a precise and successful treatment plan.

Functional assessments and detailed anatomical information are provided by diagnostic imaging and other diagnostic tools, which are essential to the chiropractic care process. When combined with the results of physical examinations, these tools enable chiropractors to accurately diagnose musculoskeletal conditions and customize treatment plans to address the root causes of pain and dysfunction.

CREATING PRACTICAL THERAPY OBJECTIVES

Establishing achievable outcomes based on the nature of the condition, the assessment findings, and the patient's health goals is a collaborative process between the chiropractor and the patient. Setting realistic treatment goals is an integral part of the initial chiropractic consultation, as it sets clear objectives for the patient's recovery and improvement.

Reducing pain and inflammation, increasing joint mobility, correcting spinal alignment, improving overall musculoskeletal function, and fostering long-term wellness are just a few of the possible treatment objectives. The chiropractor creates a treatment plan for each patient by defining clear expectations and deadlines, which keeps everyone involved and transparent.

By fostering a positive therapeutic experience that is centered on enhancing the patient's quality of life and regaining optimal musculoskeletal health, chiropractors enable patients to take an active role in their healing process and encourage them to follow prescribed treatment regimens.

CHAPTER FIVE

TECHNIQUES FOR ADJUSTMENTS IN CHIROPRACTIC

THE PURPOSE AND DEFINITION OF CHIROPRACTIC ADJUSTMENTS

Spinal manipulations, another name for chiropractic adjustments, are therapeutic procedures used by chiropractors to correct misalignments in the spine or other joints.

The main objectives of these procedures are to improve mobility, relieve pain, and enhance the overall function of the musculoskeletal system; by applying controlled force to joints that have become restricted in their range of motion, chiropractors hope to optimize nervous system function, reduce inflammation, and promote healing of injured tissues. The foundation of chiropractic adjustments is the idea that when the body's musculoskeletal structure is properly aligned, it can heal itself without the need for surgery or medication.

Techniques used can vary depending on the patient's condition, preferences, and the chiropractor's expertise, ensuring a personalized approach to treatment. Chiropractic adjustments involve precise movements that are typically applied manually or with specialized instruments.

Each adjustment is customized to the unique needs of the patient, focusing on areas of the spine or joints that are dysfunctional or causing discomfort. By restoring normal joint function, chiropractors help relieve pressure on surrounding tissues, reduce pain, and improve overall physical well-being.

Patients frequently report immediate relief or improvement in symptoms following adjustments, though multiple sessions may be required for long-lasting results. Knowledge of the objectives and techniques of chiropractic adjustments can empower people to make educated decisions about their health and seek appropriate care for their individual needs.

Back pain, neck pain, headaches, and joint stiffness are among the conditions for which people seek chiropractic adjustments.

VARIOUS ADJUSTMENT TECHNIQUE TYPES

To restore normal movement and alignment to misaligned joints, chiropractors use a variety of adjustment techniques that are customized to the needs and preferences of their patients. One such technique is the diversified technique, which is a widely used and adaptable method that involves applying a quick thrust with the hands of the chiropractor to the misaligned joint.

Another method is the activator method, which uses a small, spring-loaded device called an activator to deliver a gentle impulse to the targeted area, enabling chiropractors to make accurate adjustments without using force. Patients who may find manual adjustments uncomfortable or who have particular conditions that call for a gentler approach are frequently candidates for the activator method.

With a focus on targeted correction and improved joint function, chiropractors employing the Gonstead technique identify specific misalignments by carefully analyzing X-rays and performing physical examinations. The method emphasizes a thorough assessment and individualized treatment plan based on each patient's unique spinal biomechanics.

Every adjustment technique has pros and cons that vary based on the patient's condition, degree of comfort, and the chiropractor's experience. Patients can choose the best approach for their chiropractic care by talking with their healthcare provider about these options, which will help to promote efficient treatment and the best possible results.

PRACTICAL DISPLAY OF ADJUSTMENT PROCESSES

To determine the proper technique and force for an adjustment, the chiropractor first assesses the patient's spine or affected joint to find areas of misalignment or restricted movement.

The chiropractor uses palpation and occasionally imaging techniques like X-rays to pinpoint the exact areas that need to be adjusted.

The patient may lie face down, on their side, or sit upright depending on the area being treated. Once the targeted joint has been identified, the patient is positioned on a specialized adjusting table or chair designed to optimize access to the spine or joint.

The chiropractor then applies controlled force using their hands or a specialized instrument to the targeted joint to restore normal movement and alignment.

To reduce pain, improve mobility, and enhance overall joint function, the adjustment process itself entails a quick, controlled thrust or gentle pressure on the affected joint. This is often accompanied by a popping or cracking sound as gases are released from the joint capsule—a normal and harmless occurrence. The adjustment process is repeated as necessary for each identified area of concern.

Knowing the practical steps involved in chiropractic adjustments can allay fears and give patients the confidence to actively participate in their treatment plan for the best possible outcome. Patients usually experience immediate relief or improvement in symptoms following adjustments, though mild soreness or discomfort may occur initially, which usually resolves quickly.

Chiropractors may also provide guidance on posture, exercises, and ergonomic modifications to support ongoing spinal health and prevent future issues.

SAFETY OBSERVATIONS WHEN MAKING CHANGES

Before beginning treatment, chiropractors thoroughly evaluate the patient's medical history, current state of health, and any conditions that may affect the safety or outcome of adjustments. Adjustments made by licensed, trained chiropractors are generally safe. However, some safety precautions must be taken to ensure effectiveness and reduce potential risks associated with adjustments.

To achieve therapeutic benefits without causing harm, chiropractors use precise techniques and controlled force to target joints during adjustments. Patients may experience mild soreness or discomfort after adjustments, but this is normal and usually goes away on its own.

Serious complications, like nerve compression or aggravated pain, are rare but can happen, emphasizing the need for proper assessment and technique by qualified practitioners.

To ensure safe and effective care, chiropractors prioritize patient safety by tailoring treatment plans to each patient's unique needs and conditions. Patients with osteoporosis, spinal abnormalities, or other specific health concerns, may modify treatment approaches or adjust techniques. Patients and chiropractors are encouraged to communicate openly about any discomfort, concerns, or changes in symptoms to maximize treatment outcomes and maintain a collaborative approach to healthcare.

By following established safety protocols and guidelines, chiropractors support their patients' long-term wellness and foster a positive treatment experience. Patients who are aware of the safety considerations during adjustments are better able to make informed decisions about their care and take an active role in maintaining the health of their spines.

SUBSEQUENT CARE FOLLOWING ADJUSTMENTS

To maximize treatment results and support long-term spinal health, patients may benefit from particular follow-up care strategies after receiving adjustments from a chiropractor. In addition to adjustments, chiropractors frequently offer advice on posture correction, ergonomic changes, and therapeutic exercises to support and enhance spinal alignment.

Following adjustments, patients may feel immediate relief or improvement in their symptoms; however, to maintain the health of their spine and avoid future issues, it is usually advised that patients receive ongoing care. Regular follow-up visits to a chiropractor can help address underlying issues, lower the risk of spinal misalignments, and support overall musculoskeletal function. The frequency of these visits varies depending on the patient, the goals of treatment, and the severity of the condition being addressed.

To support spinal health, in addition to making adjustments to the spine, practitioners may also suggest lifestyle changes like eating a healthy diet, exercising regularly, and using safe lifting techniques. These proactive steps lead to long-lasting gains in flexibility, mobility, and general well-being, which in turn improves the efficacy of chiropractic care over time.

Open communication between patients and their chiropractors regarding any changes in symptoms, concerns, or progress is encouraged. This collaborative approach allows for necessary modifications to the treatment plan and fosters individualized care that is customized to each patient's unique health goals. Patients can optimize the long-term benefits of chiropractic adjustments and experience improved spinal function by implementing follow-up care strategies into their routines.

CHAPTER SIX

ADJUNCTIVE THERAPIES IN CHIROPRACTIC MEDICINE

SYNOPSIS OF COMPLEMENTARY MEDICINE

Complementary therapies are essential to the treatment process because they improve patient outcomes and promote overall well-being. Therapeutic exercises are basic components that target specific musculoskeletal issues that are found during assessments conducted by chiropractors. Patients can gradually rehabilitate injured or weak areas by following prescribed movements and stretches, which can help prevent future injuries and promote long-term recovery.

Another important tool used in chiropractic care is ultrasound therapy, which is especially useful for reducing pain and inflammation. Ultrasound therapy uses high-frequency sound waves to penetrate deeply into tissues, increasing circulation and hastening the healing process.

This non-invasive treatment modality is frequently incorporated into chiropractic care to lessen muscle spasms, improve tissue repair, and increase overall joint mobility. By learning about these therapies, those new to chiropractic care can appreciate their roles in improving patient outcomes and increasing possibilities for treatment.

HOW CHIROPRACTIC ADJUSTMENTS ARE SUPPORTED BY COMPLEMENTARY THERAPIES

When combined with chiropractic adjustments, therapeutic exercises help stabilizes the spine and surrounding muscles. This synergy not only reinforces the benefits of manual adjustments but also extends the therapeutic effects beyond the chiropractic session.

Patients learn corrective exercises that strengthen supportive muscles, reducing the likelihood of recurring misalignments and promoting spinal health over time. Complementary therapies are supportive measures for chiropractic adjustments that enhance the effectiveness and sustainability of spinal alignments.

A beginner in chiropractic care gains insight into these synergistic relationships, understanding how combining therapies can optimize patient comfort and therapeutic outcomes. Ultrasound therapy complements chiropractic adjustments by addressing soft tissue injuries and inflammation. Before adjustments, ultrasound treatments can relax tight muscles and increase circulation to the affected area, making adjustments more comfortable and effective. Following an adjustment, ultrasound continues to support healing by reducing swelling and promoting tissue repair.

ADVANTAGES AND DRAWBACKS OF EVERY THERAPY

Enhancing flexibility, strengthening muscles, and stabilizing joints are just a few of the advantages that come with therapeutic exercises. These exercises are customized to each person and target particular areas of weakness or imbalance that are found during chiropractic examinations. On the other hand, if exercises are done poorly or unsupervised, they can exacerbate pre-existing conditions, so it's important for newcomers to closely adhere to recommended exercise regimens and consult with chiropractors to optimize benefits and minimize risks.

Ultrasound therapy is a non-invasive, well-tolerated treatment that reduces pain, inflammation, and muscle spasms through deep tissue penetration. It can also speed up the healing process for patients with musculoskeletal injuries. However, despite its benefits, there are some conditions where ultrasound therapy is not appropriate, such as acute infections or malignancies where deep heat application could be dangerous. Those new to the field of chiropractic care will learn to identify these risks and how to safely and effectively integrate ultrasound into their treatments.

COMBINING THERAPIES FOR ALL-INCLUSIVE CARE

To fully address the complex needs of patients, effective chiropractic care frequently combines multiple therapies. For example, combining therapeutic exercises with chiropractic adjustments results in a holistic approach that targets both spinal alignment and muscular support. This integrated approach improves treatment outcomes by addressing the underlying causes of musculoskeletal dysfunction and promoting overall wellness. Treatment plans can also benefit from the addition of ultrasound therapy, which can reduce pain and inflammation, speed up recovery, and improve patient comfort.

Chiropractic care novices learn the art of treatment planning, balancing various therapies to optimize patient outcomes while ensuring safety and effectiveness. This comprehensive approach not only enhances clinical results but also strengthens patient trust and satisfaction in chiropractic care.

Chiropractors can provide individualized treatment plans that are tailored to each patient's unique condition and goals by strategically integrating complementary therapies.

TAILORED CARE PROGRAMS

The cornerstone of effective chiropractic care is personalized treatment plans, which guarantee that therapies are customized to meet the unique needs and health goals of each patient. Individualized exercises address strengths, weaknesses, and mobility challenges, promoting targeted rehabilitation and injury prevention. By incorporating lifestyle factors and patient preferences into treatment planning, chiropractors enable patients to actively participate in their recovery, fostering long-term health benefits and adherence to treatment protocols.

The location and severity of musculoskeletal injuries determine the personalized nature of ultrasound therapy, and treatment parameters are adjusted to maximize therapeutic outcomes.

Chiropractors evaluate how their patients respond to ultrasound treatments, adjusting protocols as necessary to account for changes in the patient's condition or progress in healing. This personalized approach not only improves the efficacy of treatment but also fosters patient comfort and confidence in chiropractic care. Newcomers discover the value of being flexible in treatment planning and modifying protocols to suit changing patient needs and conditions.

CHAPTER SEVEN
CONDITIONS CHIROPRACTORS TREAT
TREATMENT FOR COMMON MUSCULOSKELETAL CONDITIONS

Chiropractic adjustments are intended to realign the spine and relieve pressure on nerves, muscles, and joints, promoting natural healing and improved function. Back pain, which includes problems such as lower back pain, upper back pain, and spinal misalignments that can cause discomfort and limited mobility, is one of the most common musculoskeletal conditions treated by chiropractors. Another common condition they treat is neck pain, which is frequently brought on by poor posture, stress, or injuries.

Other musculoskeletal conditions treated include sports injuries, such as sprains, strains, and tendonitis, where chiropractic adjustments aid in speeding up recovery and preventing recurrent injuries.

By addressing these conditions holistically, chiropractic care aims to enhance overall wellness and quality of life for patients. Joint pain, such as that in the shoulders, hips, and knees, can also be caused by repetitive movements, overuse, or injuries. These treatments focus on restoring joint mobility and reducing inflammation through manual adjustments and therapeutic exercises.

CHIROPRACTIC BENEFITS FOR PARTICULAR CONDITIONS

Beyond musculoskeletal pain, chiropractic care has been shown to have substantial benefits for several conditions. For example, it has been demonstrated to effectively reduce headaches, including tension headaches and migraines, by reducing muscular tension and improving spinal alignment.

Following regular adjustments, patients frequently report fewer and less severe headaches. Additionally, chiropractic care is effective for treating sciatica, a painful condition caused by compression of the sciatic nerve. By using targeted adjustments and therapeutic exercises, chiropractors can relieve pressure on the sciatic nerve, thereby reducing pain and enhancing mobility.

Chiropractic adjustments help patients manage symptoms and improve their overall quality of life. The holistic approach to chiropractic care emphasizes not only pain relief but also enhancing the body's natural healing abilities and promoting long-term wellness. Patients often report improved sleep, decreased reliance on pain medications, and increased energy levels as a result of receiving customized care. Additionally, chiropractic adjustments have been found beneficial for managing conditions such as fibromyalgia and arthritis.

EVIDENCE-BASED CHIROPRACTIC CARE METHODS

Chiropractors receive extensive training to diagnose conditions accurately and create individualized treatment plans based on the most recent clinical guidelines and research findings. Evidence-based practices, which prioritize patient safety and effectiveness, are the foundation of chiropractic care. Techniques like spinal manipulation, mobilization, and therapeutic exercises are supported by scientific research demonstrating their efficacy in treating musculoskeletal conditions and improving spinal function.

Studies show that adjustments made by chiropractors can result in decreased pain, increased range of motion, and improved physical function in patients with a variety of musculoskeletal disorders. Evidence-based chiropractic care includes lifestyle changes, patient education, and preventive techniques to enable people to take charge of their health.

CASE STUDIES SHOWING EFFECTIVE THERAPIES

Case studies offer strong evidence of the efficacy of chiropractic care in treating a variety of musculoskeletal conditions.

For instance, a case study may describe how a patient with chronic lower back pain was able to achieve significant pain relief and increased mobility after receiving therapeutic exercises and adjustments from a chiropractor. These studies also highlight customized treatment regimens that are based on the individual needs of each patient and the severity of their condition.

Case studies also highlight the holistic approach of chiropractic care, which frequently incorporates nutritional counseling, ergonomic recommendations, and lifestyle modifications to optimize treatment outcomes. An additional case study might center on a patient who experienced recurrent migraines and found relief through chiropractic care aimed at correcting spinal misalignments and reducing muscular tension in the neck and shoulders. Such success stories highlight the transformative impact of chiropractic adjustments on patients' daily lives, emphasizing not just symptom management but also long-term wellness goals.

THE VALUE OF CONTINUOUS CHIROPRACTIC CARE FOR LONG-TERM ILLNESSES

In patients with long-term musculoskeletal disorders, regular adjustments from a chiropractor are essential to controlling symptoms and averting flare-ups. While medications offer short-term pain relief, regular adjustments from a chiropractor address the root causes of chronic pain, such as joint dysfunction or spinal misalignments. Over time, patients can improve their mobility, experience less pain, and feel better overall.

To support long-term health outcomes for patients with chronic conditions, chiropractors emphasize proactive maintenance and preventive care strategies. Examples of this approach include regular spinal assessments, customized exercise regimens, and ergonomic advice to minimize strain on affected joints and muscles. Patients benefit from a collaborative relationship with their chiropractor,

CHAPTER EIGHT
THE RISKS AND SAFETY OF CHIROPRACTIC CARE

RECOGNIZING THE SAFETY PROFILE OF CHIROPRACTIC ADJUSTMENT METHODS

A variety of techniques are available in chiropractic care that are intended to relieve musculoskeletal problems and enhance general health. Patients and practitioners need to know the safety profile of these techniques, as most chiropractors use spinal adjustments, mobilization techniques, and adjunctive therapies like ultrasound or electrical stimulation. These procedures are safe as long as they are carried out by professionals with the necessary training, but risks can occur if they are not customized to the patient's specific needs or if underlying health conditions are disregarded.

To ensure patient safety, chiropractors undergo extensive training to assess patient suitability for treatment and adjust techniques accordingly.

Patients considering chiropractic care should be aware of potential side effects, such as temporary soreness, stiffness, or mild headaches following adjustments. Serious complications, though rare, may include herniated discs or worsening of existing spinal conditions if adjustments are performed improperly. Regular communication between patient and practitioner is essential to address any concerns and effectively monitor progress.

The safety profile of chiropractic techniques can help patients make informed decisions about their healthcare journey, ensuring personalized and effective treatment plans under professional guidance. For those who are new to chiropractic care, investigating the credentials of practitioners, seeking referrals, and having an open discussion about health histories with providers can enhance safety and optimize treatment outcomes.

HAZARDS ASSOCIATED WITH ADJUSTMENTS IN CHIROPRACTIC

Chiropractic adjustments involve applying controlled force to joints, primarily the spine, to improve mobility and alleviate pain. While adjustments are generally safe, there are some risks to take into account to make an informed treatment decision. Common risks include soreness or discomfort immediately after treatment, which usually goes away within hours to days. Less common risks include herniated discs, nerve compression, or strokes, especially in patients with pre-existing vascular conditions.

To minimize risks and maximize treatment benefits, chiropractors use specialized training and diagnostic tools. Before making any adjustments, they must conduct thorough assessments to determine the patient's suitability and identify any contraindications. Patients who suffer from severe osteoporosis, spinal cord compression, or certain autoimmune conditions may need to undergo alternative therapies or modifications to traditional chiropractic techniques.

Patients can reduce risks by being transparent with their chiropractors, sharing medical histories, and reporting any unusual symptoms as soon as possible. Selecting a skilled practitioner who puts patient safety first and adheres to evidence-based practices is crucial. Patients can pursue effective musculoskeletal care that meets their needs with confidence if they are aware of the possible risks associated with chiropractic adjustments and have an informed conversation with healthcare providers.

PRECAUTIONS FOR PATIENT POPULATIONS AT HIGH RISK

Chiropractors customize treatment plans for high-risk patients, such as elderly patients, pregnant women, patients with severe osteoporosis, and patients with compromised immune systems, using gentle techniques and avoiding high-impact adjustments that could exacerbate underlying conditions. These measures are necessary to ensure patient safety and optimize treatment outcomes.

Patients who are elderly or have autoimmune disorders, for example, may benefit from low-force adjustments or mobilization techniques to improve joint mobility without running the risk of fractures or tissue injury. Chiropractic care is frequently sought by pregnant women to relieve pregnancy-related discomforts, such as back pain, using specially designed tables and techniques that safely accommodate different stages of pregnancy.

Specialists in the field of chiropractic care are trained to identify contraindications and modify treatment plans to accommodate a wide range of patient needs compassionately. Clear lines of communication between patients and providers guarantee that concerns are promptly addressed, fostering team decision-making in the medical field. By adhering to precautions specific to high-risk groups, chiropractors maintain patient safety while providing efficient musculoskeletal care that improves overall health.

HOW TO PICK A REPUTABLE CHIROPRACTOR

Choosing a qualified chiropractor is essential for safe and successful treatment outcomes. Start by looking up the credentials of practitioners, confirming their license, and seeing if they belong to any respectable professional organizations. Qualified chiropractors go through a rigorous educational and clinical training program that emphasizes musculoskeletal health and customized therapeutic techniques for each patient.

Consider the following when evaluating chiropractors: Look for practitioners who prioritize informed consent, and discuss potential risks, benefits, and expected outcomes before initiating care. Personal recommendations from trusted healthcare providers or friends can offer valuable insights into the reputations and treatment approaches of these practitioners.

Inquire about specific techniques used, treatment philosophies, and success rates with comparable conditions during initial consultations. Evaluate the cleanliness of the clinic, patient comfort, and compliance with equipment and hygiene standards. Reputable chiropractors welcome questions regarding their training, methods of treatment, and continued education to stay up to date with the latest developments in musculoskeletal care.

Patients can confidently begin a collaborative healthcare path aimed at achieving optimal musculoskeletal wellness and enhanced quality of life by choosing a trained chiropractor who cultivates trust and transparency.

LEGAL AND MORAL ISSUES IN THE PRACTICE OF CHIROPRACTIC MEDICINE

Chiropractic professionals adhere to state licensure requirements, maintain competence through continuing education and regulatory compliance, and operate within legal and ethical frameworks designed to protect patient welfare and uphold professional standards. Ethical principles govern interactions with patients, emphasizing honesty, respect for autonomy, and confidentiality in healthcare settings.

Chiropractors prioritize patient safety by performing thorough examinations, diagnosing conditions within the scope of practice, and referring patients to appropriate healthcare providers when necessary. They also engage in comprehensive assessments to determine patient suitability for treatment, ensuring informed consent and respecting individual preferences. Transparent communication fosters trusting relationships, empowering patients to make decisions about their care.

Chiropractors are committed to truthfulness in marketing materials, avoiding misleading statements or unsubstantiated promises of cure. They uphold patient rights to privacy and informed choice, maintaining confidentiality of medical records and respecting cultural or religious beliefs affecting healthcare decisions.

CHAPTER NINE

COMBINING CHIROPRACTIC THERAPY WITH OTHER MEDICAL SPECIALTIES

WORKING COOPERATIVELY WITH PHYSICIANS AND SPECIALISTS

Chiropractors frequently collaborate with physicians, orthopedists, physical therapists, and other specialists to develop integrated treatment plans tailored to individual patient conditions. This teamwork ensures that patients receive holistic care that takes into account both spinal health and overall wellness.

In modern healthcare practices, collaboration between chiropractors and medical doctors, as well as other specialists, plays a crucial role in providing comprehensive patient care. This collaborative approach leverages the expertise of each healthcare professional to address the multifaceted needs of patients.

Clear communication and mutual respect are the foundations of effective collaboration between healthcare providers. Chiropractors and medical doctors work together to provide complementary treatments that improve therapeutic outcomes and patient satisfaction. They collaborate by exchanging patient histories, diagnostic results, and treatment plans, which helps to understand the patient's overall health context and guarantees that all aspects of their care are coordinated and optimized.

Additionally, collaborative approaches create a learning environment where medical professionals can share expertise and knowledge. By working together, doctors and chiropractors enhance patient care while also advancing integrative healthcare practices. This continuous communication allows chiropractors to stay current on medical advancements and evidence-based practices and incorporate them into their treatment protocols.

MULTIDISCIPLINARY COMMUNICATION'S SIGNIFICANCE

When it comes to ensuring that all healthcare providers involved in a patient's care are informed and on the same page regarding treatment goals, interdisciplinary communication is crucial in integrative healthcare settings where chiropractors work alongside a variety of specialists.

It entails sharing pertinent patient information, discussing treatment goals, and coordinating interventions to achieve optimal health outcomes. By utilizing the expertise of other healthcare professionals, interdisciplinary communication allows chiropractors to address complex health conditions.

Effective communication channels enable smooth transitions between various stages of care, such as initial assessment and diagnosis, treatment implementation, and follow-up. For instance, prompt referrals to suitable specialists are made possible by clear communication channels when a chiropractor determines that a patient requires further diagnostic testing or specialized medical evaluation. This proactive approach guarantees that patients receive thorough and on-time care, minimizing delays in diagnosis and treatment.

Moreover, interdisciplinary communication fosters a patient-centered approach to healthcare, wherein chiropractors and other healthcare providers empower patients to make educated decisions about their health by involving them in discussions about their care plans and treatment options. This collaborative decision-making process improves patient satisfaction and treatment compliance, which in turn leads to improved health outcomes and quality of life.

WHEN TO SEND PATIENTS TO DIFFERENT MEDICAL PROFESSIONALS

Chiropractic professionals working in integrative health settings need to know when to refer patients to other healthcare providers. Referrals are required when patients need treatments, diagnostic procedures, or specialized medical interventions that fall outside the purview of chiropractic care. Depending on the complexity of the patient's condition and the need for interdisciplinary collaboration, chiropractors should think about referring patients to medical doctors, orthopedists, neurologists, physical therapists, or other specialists.

Suspected fractures, neurological symptoms (e.g., severe radiating pain, numbness), and systemic health issues requiring medical management are common referral reasons. Patients with complex musculoskeletal disorders or chronic conditions may benefit from multidisciplinary evaluation and treatment planning. Effective communication between receiving healthcare providers and chiropractors is crucial in the coordination of referrals.

A coordinated approach that improves patient safety increases treatment efficacy, and supports comprehensive care delivery in integrative health settings is necessary for chiropractors to maintain continuity of care. These referrals should be made on a timely basis and based on clinical judgment to ensure that patients receive the appropriate care without needless delays.

CHIROPRACTIC'S PLACE IN INTEGRATIVE HEALTH ENVIRONMENTS

Chiropractors use manual techniques, spinal adjustments, and therapeutic exercises to improve joint mobility, relieve pain, and enhance physical function.

Because chiropractic care focuses on spinal health, neuromuscular function, and overall wellness, it plays a significant role in integrative health settings. In integrative settings, chiropractors collaborate with medical doctors and specialists to provide complementary treatments that address the underlying causes of musculoskeletal conditions and promote holistic healing.

A comprehensive approach to patient care is made possible by the integration of chiropractic care into multidisciplinary practices. In this approach, patients receive personalized treatment plans that take into account the connection between the musculoskeletal system and overall health.

In addition to treating acute injuries and chronic conditions, this integrative approach also supports long-term wellness strategies and preventive care. Chiropractors work in collaboration with primary care physicians, physical therapists, and other healthcare professionals.

Additionally, by concentrating on spinal alignment and nerve function, chiropractors seek to maximize biomechanical integrity and restore balance to the body's musculoskeletal system. This proactive approach to health maintenance and rehabilitation is in line with the objectives of integrative healthcare, which emphasize patient-centered care and collaborative treatment modalities. Furthermore, chiropractic care helps to manage pain and functional limitations associated with a variety of health conditions, including headaches, sports injuries, neck pain, and back pain.

PATIENT INSTRUCTION REGARDING COMBINATION THERAPY METHODS

Patient education includes explaining the role of chiropractic care in managing musculoskeletal conditions, its benefits as part of an integrated treatment plan, and how it complements conventional medical interventions. By empowering patients with knowledge about their treatment options, chiropractors promote active participation in their healthcare decisions and enhance treatment adherence.

Combined treatment approaches are important topics to educate patients about in integrative healthcare settings where chiropractors collaborate with other healthcare providers.

Chiropractors educate patients on the biomechanical effects of spinal misalignments, the significance of posture and ergonomics, and lifestyle modifications that support musculoskeletal health. This educational process fosters realistic expectations about treatment outcomes and encourages patients to take proactive steps in managing their health. Patients benefit from understanding the principles of chiropractic care, including spinal adjustments, soft tissue therapies, and rehabilitative exercises.

Furthermore, patient education dispels any doubts or fears regarding chiropractic care and how it works with other medical specialties. By answering concerns about safety, effectiveness, and collaborative treatment, chiropractors establish rapport and trust with their patients. This open communication allows for shared decision-making and motivates patients to take an active role in their recovery, which improves treatment compliance and promotes long-term wellness.

To provide comprehensive patient care, better treatment outcomes, and increased patient satisfaction, integrating chiropractic care with other medical practices in an integrative setting necessitates effective collaboration, interdisciplinary communication, prompt referrals, a defined role for chiropractic within the healthcare team, and patient education on combined treatment approaches.

CHAPTER TEN

CHANGES IN LIFESTYLE FOR SPINAL HEALTH

THE VALUE OF ERGONOMICS AND POSTURE

Proper posture is essential for preserving spinal health and avoiding pain or injury. It keeps your spine in alignment, which lessens the strain on your muscles and ligaments. Whether you're sitting, standing, or moving, good posture supports the natural curves of your spine. To maintain proper posture, keep your shoulders back, your chin parallel to the floor, and your spine neutral. Slouching or hunching forward will eventually cause muscle imbalances and back pain.

Optimizing your workspace for ergonomic comfort can lower your risk of repetitive strain injuries and improve your overall spinal health. For example, you can adjust the height of your chair so that your feet rest flat on the floor and your knees are at a right angle; place your computer screen at eye level to prevent neck strain; and use ergonomic accessories like lumbar support cushions to maintain the natural curve of your lower back. Ergonomics is a critical factor in promoting good posture, especially in home and workplace environments.

Maintaining good posture is a habit that improves your overall well-being and quality of life. It is important to incorporate these practices into your daily life for long-term spinal health. Whether you're standing in a line or sitting at a desk, doing so guarantees that your spine is correctly aligned and supported, which lowers the risk of developing spinal conditions or chronic back pain.

TIPS FOR CREATING AN ERGONOMIC WORK AND HOME ENVIRONMENT

Establishing an ergonomic workspace is essential to avoiding back strain and injury. Begin by selecting a chair that provides adequate lumbar support and height adjustment. Arrange your desk and computer monitor so that your elbows are at a 90-degree angle and your screen is at eye level. If necessary, use a footrest to support your feet and preserve blood flow in your legs. Finally, take frequent breaks to stretch and shift positions to prevent sitting for extended periods.

Use ergonomic tools and equipment at home: Use long-handled gardening tools or ergonomic kitchen utensils to reduce strain; when watching television or reading, support your lower back with cushions or pillows to maintain a comfortable sitting position; and when lifting heavy objects, bend your knees and keep your back straight to avoid straining your spine.

You may build surroundings at home and at work that support spinal health and lower the risk of injury by using these ergonomic ideas. Small changes over time can have a big impact on your comfort and overall well-being.

INCLUDING STRETCHING AND EXERCISE PROGRAMS

Maintaining spinal health and flexibility requires regular exercise and stretching. Exercises that target the core muscles supporting your spine, like yoga, Pilates, or swimming, help to stabilize the spine and improve posture, which lowers the risk of back pain and injury. You should also include stretching exercises in your daily routine to improve your flexibility and release tension in the muscles that surround your spine.

To strengthen and stabilize the spine, concentrate on exercises that work the back, abdomen, and hips. For instance, practice planks or bird-dog exercises to strengthen the muscles that support the spine. Similarly, hamstring stretches and cat-cow stretches can help to increase flexibility and decrease stiffness in the legs and back. Make time each day or week to incorporate these routines into your schedule to experience better overall health and spinal health.

Consistency is key to maintaining spinal health and enjoying a pain-free lifestyle. Start slowly and gradually increase the intensity of your workouts to avoid strain or overexertion. By prioritizing exercise and stretching, you support the natural alignment of your spine and reduce the risk of spinal conditions or injuries.

DIETARY SUGGESTIONS TO PROMOTE SPINAL HEALTH

A healthy, well-balanced diet is crucial for maintaining strong bones and supporting the structure of the spine. To guarantee that you are getting enough calcium, include foods like dairy products, leafy greens, nuts, and fortified cereals in your diet. Vitamin D, which is found in fatty fish, eggs, and sunlight exposure, aids in the body's absorption of calcium.

Consume foods high in omega-3 fatty acids, which are found in nuts and fish, and fruits and vegetables to help heal the spine by reducing inflammation.

Processed foods, sugar, and saturated fats should be avoided as they can cause weight gain and inflammation, which can worsen spinal conditions.

Water also acts as a cushion and lubricant for the joints and discs in the spine, so it's important to stay hydrated. Try to drink a lot of water throughout the day and avoid sugar-filled beverages and alcohol, which can dry the body and aggravate inflammation.

Reducing inflammation, maintaining strong bones, and promoting overall well-being are all made possible by implementing a healthy diet that promotes spinal health. It's important to keep in mind that dietary decisions affect not only your overall health and quality of life but also your spinal health.

THE EFFECTS OF STRESS MANAGEMENT STRATEGIES ON SPINAL HEALTH

Incorporating stress management techniques into your daily routine can assist to release tension and promote relaxation, reducing the risk of stress-related spinal disorders. Chronic stress can lead to muscle tension and pain in the back and neck, damaging spinal health over time.

Throughout the day, take breaks to stretch and engage in mindfulness exercises that help you focus on the present moment and release tension in the muscles surrounding your spine. Stress-related back pain can be mitigated by practicing relaxation techniques like deep breathing, meditation, or yoga, which help to calm the mind and body.

Exercise helps to release built-up tension in the muscles and promotes relaxation, which can improve overall spinal health. Incorporate enjoyable activities, like walking, dancing, or cycling, to relieve stress and support a healthy spine. Regular physical activity can lower stress levels and increase the body's production of mood-enhancing endorphins.

In addition, make sure you get enough sleep so that your body has time to recuperate and heal. Inadequate sleep can lead to higher stress levels and tense muscles, which can negatively impact spinal health. Establish a soothing evening routine and furnish your sleeping space comfortably to encourage sound sleep and enhance general health.

Remember, stress management is crucial to keeping a healthy spine and leading a pain-free lifestyle. By incorporating stress management practices into your everyday life, you may lessen the negative effects of stress on your spinal health and enhance overall well-being.

CHAPTER ELEVEN

FAQS & FREQUENTLY ASKED QUESTIONS

COMMON QUESTIONS AND ANSWERS REGARDING CHIROPRACTIC CARE

Non-invasive treatments for musculoskeletal health, with a focus on the spine, are known to be effective and safe. By correcting spinal misalignments, chiropractic adjustments have been shown to reduce pain and increase mobility, which can have a positive impact on overall health and wellness. Patients frequently ask what conditions can be treated with chiropractic care; the list includes headaches, joint problems, back and neck pain, and more. Each treatment plan is unique, with adjustments made to meet the needs of the patient. Other potential benefits include better posture and improved nerve function, which can improve overall health.

Chiropractors use precise techniques to manipulate the spine and other joints, minimizing risks.

Before treatment, they conduct thorough evaluations, including health history reviews and physical examinations, to determine the appropriateness of chiropractic care for each patient. This thorough approach helps ensure safety and effectiveness. Patients may be concerned about the popping or cracking sounds occasionally heard during adjustments. These are normal and result from the release of gas bubbles in the joints as they are realigned.

Additionally, chiropractic care often entails more than just adjustments; it may involve therapeutic exercises, nutritional advice, and ergonomic recommendations to support long-term health. Education plays a crucial role, as chiropractors empower patients with knowledge about their condition and self-care practices to enhance treatment outcomes.

By addressing common concerns through education and personalized care, chiropractors strive to optimize patient well-being and quality of life.

Patients should be aware of potential side effects, such as mild soreness or stiffness following adjustments, as these typically subside quickly and are considered a normal part of the healing process.

RESOLVING SAFETY AND EFFECTIVENESS ISSUES

Chiropractic care is often viewed with concerns regarding safety and efficacy. Safety is a top priority in chiropractic practices, and practitioners receive extensive training and education. Before beginning any treatment, chiropractors are trained to thoroughly assess patients, ensuring that adjustments are safe and appropriate. The techniques used in chiropractic care are gentle and precise, customized to the individual needs and conditions of each patient, reducing risks and improving efficacy.

Effectiveness is yet another important factor to take into account. There is research to support the use of chiropractic care for a variety of musculoskeletal conditions, such as headaches, neck pain, and back pain. Studies also show that the adjustments made by a chiropractor can enhance overall quality of life, improve spinal function, and reduce pain. Patients typically feel better after just a few sessions, though the number of treatments required varies depending on the severity of the condition and the patient's response to care.

Possible side effects from chiropractic adjustments are usually minor and infrequent. They can include minor soreness or discomfort following adjustments, which usually goes away quickly.

Serious complications are very uncommon and are usually caused by improper technique or pre-existing conditions. Patients can increase their safety by selecting a qualified chiropractor who is licensed, has good patient reviews, and is open to open communication.

WHAT TO ANTICIPATE FROM A VISIT TO THE CHIROPRACTOR

Patients can feel less anxious and more at ease during their visits to the chiropractor if they are aware of what to expect. First, the chiropractor will perform a thorough evaluation that includes a review of the patient's medical history, a physical examination, and, if needed, the ordering of diagnostic tests such as X-rays. This assessment helps the chiropractor determine the patient's condition and develop a treatment plan that addresses it. Patients are encouraged to discuss their symptoms, concerns, and treatment goals during the evaluation.

Chiropractic adjustments are manual manipulations of the spine and joints used to correct misalignments; their purpose is to restore proper joint function and alleviate pain; patients often experience immediate relief or improvement in symptoms following adjustments; however, depending on the severity of the condition, the full benefits may require multiple sessions.

Adjustments may pop or crack as gas bubbles are released from the joints; this is normal and not painful.

Patients should anticipate that their chiropractor will educate them on self-care practices, such as posture correction and ergonomic adjustments in daily activities. Regular visits may be recommended initially to monitor progress and adjust treatment plans as needed.

By being prepared, patients can actively participate in their recovery and achieve optimal health outcomes through chiropractic care. In addition to adjustments, chiropractic care may include other therapeutic interventions like soft tissue therapies, rehabilitative exercises, and ergonomic recommendations. These complementary treatments support the healing process and help prevent future injuries.

HOW TO LOCATE A TRUSTWORTHY CHIROPRACTOR

Seeking recommendations from medical professionals, friends, or family members who have had good experiences with chiropractic care is a good place to start. Online reviews and testimonials can also give you insight into the reputation and patient satisfaction of chiropractors. Look for chiropractors who are licensed and accredited by reputable chiropractic associations, as this guarantees they meet high standards of education and practice. Finding a reputable chiropractor requires research and careful consideration to ensure quality care and positive outcomes.

Make sure the chiropractor you choose has the training and experience necessary to treat your particular condition. For example, some chiropractors specialize in treating sports injuries, while others treat pediatric patients or manage chronic pain. It's important to find a chiropractor whose knowledge and skills match your needs and health objectives. Make an appointment for a consultation or initial visit so you can meet the chiropractor in person and talk about your concerns, treatment options, and anticipated results. This meeting also gives you a chance to evaluate the chiropractor's professionalism, communication style, and willingness to answer your questions.

Ultimately, trust your gut and select a chiropractor who listens to your concerns, respects your preferences, and places a high priority on your health and well-being. During the consultation, take note of the clinic's cleanliness, organization, and general atmosphere. A well-kept and welcoming environment reflects the chiropractor's commitment to patient care and comfort. Ask about the treatment techniques used and any additional services offered, such as nutritional counseling or rehabilitation exercises. Transparency regarding treatment costs, insurance coverage, and payment options is also important to avoid unforeseen expenses.

SOURCES OF ADDITIONAL DATA AND ASSISTANCE

Obtaining additional information and assistance from credible sources can improve your comprehension of chiropractic care and assist you in making well-informed decisions regarding your health. To begin, look into respectable websites and publications recommended by chiropractic associations, like the American Chiropractic Association or the International Chiropractors Association. These groups offer insightful information about chiropractic principles, available treatments, and patient testimonials, enabling you to gain more knowledge about the advantages and efficacy of chiropractic care.

Consider attending seminars or webinars hosted by chiropractors or healthcare professionals to expand your knowledge and ask questions directly to experts in the field. Many chiropractors also offer educational materials and workshops that explain common musculoskeletal conditions, treatment techniques, and preventive care strategies. These resources empower patients to take an active role in their health and well-being by providing practical tips for maintaining spinal health and preventing injuries.

Social media platforms and healthcare apps may also feature chiropractic professionals sharing educational content, patient success stories, and updates on advancements in spinal care. Online forums and support groups can connect you with individuals who have undergone chiropractic treatment or are considering it. Peer discussions can offer insightful information, firsthand accounts, and recommendations for locating reputable chiropractors in your area.

Finally, by using a variety of resources, you can learn everything there is to know about chiropractic care and proceed with confidence on your path to better spinal health and general well-being.

www.ingramcontent.com/pod-product-compliance
Lightning Source LLC
Chambersburg PA
CBHW071835210526
45479CB00001B/147